The Rich Tapestry of Life

Synchronicity: We are all connected.

Vol 7

Extract from the original book,

'A Glimpse in a Transient Zone'

Jo Eaton.

Copyright.

Disclaimer.

The author of this book does not dispense medical advice or prescribe the use of any technique as a form of treatment for physical or medical problems without the advice of a physician, either directly or indirectly. The intent of the author is only to offer information of a general nature to help you in your quest for emotional and spiritual well-being. In the event you use any of the information in this book for yourself, which Is your constitutional right, the author and the publisher assume no responsibility for your actions.

In order to protect identity, I have changed the names of some of the characters within many of the stories.

Contents

Chapter 1

The Hidden Intelligence Guiding You

Throughout my journey, I have been aware of synchronistic events which have helped me on my way. It may have been a stranger entering my life, a random leaflet pushed through my front door, or even a book beckoning me from the shelves of a book shop. There are many ways of being 'directed' or even receiving help with your aims in life, but it is important to be vigilant in looking out for such messages. I will give you just one example of such a happening in my life:

I had always wanted to be a full-time professional artist, but once I had completed my Degree, I had to look for a regular income, in order to support my three children through University. Hence, I put my desires on hold and trained to be a teacher.

After several years teaching, I discovered there were only a few Universities who offered a part-time MA course in my chosen area, one being at Camden in London. Although by this time, I had two sons at University and another child at home, I was able to commit to the part-time course available and so notified my employer of my intentions. However, once the school time-table had been published, I found my reduced hours had been spread across the whole week, with a refusal to negotiate any further. This dashed my plans again to follow my dream.

It was a further five more years I waited, for when synchronicity entered into my life regarding my artwork. My husband found a leaflet which had been pushed through the letterbox, announcing a list of new MA part-time courses were being offered at my local University, one being in my chosen area. I could hardly believe my luck because this would be by far more convenient for me, not having to travel and stay over in London. Needless to say, while still teaching, I simultaneously thoroughly enjoyed studying on my MA Degree, which opened even more doors to help me on my way.

Positive thoughts attract synchronicity, with good outcomes and yet negative thoughts, driven by fear, should be dismissed and cleared as soon as they come. Another positive image should be willed in your mind, as a replacement, then eventually all negative thoughts diminish. However, if you have a premonition regarding a negative event, then you need to follow your intuition, in order to avoid the situation.

Chapter 2

Be Alert to Significant Signs and Messages

Since I have become aware of this energy flow, linked with intuition, I have been constantly looking for the right people, situation or event, to help me on my way. This behaviour has often been a valuable exercise for me, bringing all sorts of events and opportunities in my life, that I would never before have considered, almost like an intuitive guidance, a confirmation that I am travelling on the right path for me. I actually feel exhilarated at those times because I know it is what I should be doing with my life and as a result, I grow and exist on a higher vibration. Other people pick up on this increased resonance, as your confidence and knowledge increases. It is also possible to see coincidences in retrospect. For example, I was making notes of my ambitions years ago, just because I could not sleep at night. I never imagined I would be turning to those journals thirty years later, but I see now, it was all a part of my life's plan.

Most events in our life contain a message of significance for us, but we also need to learn to interact with other people in a way that more messages are shared, remembering to stay centred at all times. However, it is important not to become addicted to another person because this will stunt your growth. Our aim must be open and receptive to all new varied experiences and people, in order for us to develop to our full potential.

I believe each of our previous lives have been events where we have moved towards our total advancement achieved today. I think we are a total sum of our previous experiences and with each life, we continue to slowly make progress towards enlightenment. Sometimes, we attract animals into our lives and they show up to inform us about a certain situation. It is synchronicity in action and so we must always be on the lookout for not only humans but birds and animals too, so we are able to interpret their message.

I now try to be aware of any bird who maybe singing at my window for a long time or animals unexpectedly appearing in my life because I am sure there must be some instruction for me to interpret, so we must always be vigilant.

Just recently I noticed a very large grasshopper had landed on my lounge window. He was there for at least five hours, never moving, even when closely being photographed or inspected. After researching the symbolic messages of grasshoppers, it appears to be a very fortuitous sign of good luck and prosperity. The mystery is to observe the bird or animals' way of life, in order to interpret a meaningful lesson into our present stage of development.

I have had messages for other people, which just popped into my head, not making much sense to me, but having a marked response to the listener. It was following the advice of several friends and strangers which has led me to this new venture of writing this book. It was a continuous message; one I was unable to ignore. I had no intentions to write, but to develop my ideas through my visual art work. Hopefully, I will still have the opportunity to develop this work even further since many concepts are amassing in my head, with a strong urge to create and share my ideas, such is the driving engine of creativity and intuition.

While on holiday in Italy last year, I was lounging by the hotel pool when to my right, I 'saw' a large four-pronged fork. I did not understand the significance of this dinner fork, but then I realised it was far more robust, as a garden fork.

Oh, I then realised it was for my daughter in the UK, who had just received a replacement gardening fork, because the original was damaged. On returning to the UK, I checked with my daughter and yes, she had received the gardening fork in the post exactly at the time I had visualised it.

Chapter 3

Heightened Energy Vibrations

Some of my relationships are extremely special and connected, almost spiritual. When you are within this heightened energy vibration, then this is the time when friends, or even strangers make suggestions that may help you on your way. Perhaps you are given a book or receive an unexpected phone call which may hold a magical message. It is synchronicity at its best, linking to the universal force. This has happened to me on numerous occasions, when I have followed up their suggestions, all making sense to me, even though the parted information may not have made sense to the other person.

I was aware of being in a heightened state of vibration when I was creating my healing environmental artwork. There were no restrictions or boundaries and this state of enthusiasm resonated, attracting even more energy into my life. I was living on a natural high, talking with such excitement and full of energy which dissipated onto others around me. When this happens, I know I am on the right track and following my life's purpose.

Chapter 4

Stay Open to New Ideas

It is through this wonderful synchronicity of events that helps each one of us to co-create and promote the evolution of our species. We must all stay open to new ideas and suggestions, taking a risk and following your gut reaction. This is when you are following your intuition and most probably your life's path.

I remember a very dear friend of mine, who I greatly admired and loved, giving me some valuable advice. She was very intelligent, amusing, well read, lively and extremely creative. Even in the early 60's, she was forward thinking, returning to work after raising her family, gaining promotion following successful exam results, driving a colourful sports car, with the hood down, wearing stylish clothes with such panache, silk scarf trailing in the wind. It was very rare to see a woman driving a car in this era, and more so, of being the precursor of today's modern career woman. During her eighties, she flew unaccompanied to Canada to visit her son, produced exquisite textiles, visited the theatre and organised an ex-Civil Servants Club. The lists of Greta's activities were impressive and endless while just nothing seemed to faze her. My friend was still very active in her middle nineties, when she parted some invaluable advice to me. On hearing of my invitation to travel around China, she told me to grab the chance with both hands. Always say' yes' to new opportunities coming your way, otherwise, the offers rarely come around again and you will look back with regret of not taking up such an offer. Usually, they turn out to be life changing. What wonderful 'pearls of wisdom', parting with such valuable advice.

Chapter 5

The Magic of Synchronicity

Our friend James, on a recent trip from Chile, was staying with us for a few days and so we visited the nearby National Trust property, Shrugborough Hall, near Stafford., originally owned by the British aristocratic Anson family.

Within the beautiful house, one of the upstairs rooms, was designated as an educational resource, with certain artefacts collected from around the world. A large table displayed a map of the journey of Admiral George Anson sailing around Chile, as he navigated the world in the eighteenth century.

James was very interested and surprised at this 'find' because when in Chile, he teaches English and so this excellent resource would prove to be a very useful teaching aid for when he returned home.

Following this interesting tour of the Hall and a lovely walk around the extensive grounds, we were in the courtyard when I suggested we call into the second-hand book shop. While inside the shop, James mentioned he was shortly visiting Ecuador on business, just as he then found one solitary travel book on Ecuador. I then looked down onto a much lower shelf, only to find a different travel book, 'The Lonely Planet Book of Ecuador'. Both books were extremely cheap and James was rather taken aback and delighted at such find.

On our way out of the shop, there was another table, scattered with a variety of books, on various topics and yet, on top of this pile was a certain new novel my friend was intending to buy for his partner while still on holiday in the UK. He was staring in disbelief at such a coincidence, but after I had bought this book for a nominal fee, I explained about the delights of synchronicity.

I think James is starting to move towards being open minded about holistic happenings, after hearing a few more stories.

About five years ago, my son, who emigrated to Australia seventeen years ago, entered and won an open camp cooking competition. A few weeks later, Mike and I attended our local fete, in a small West Midlands town in the UK. Browsing through the books on the charity stall, we chanced upon a cook book for open camp cooking in the Australian outback in the 1800's. The book was written in my son's local small gold-digging town called Bendigo. I was so taken aback at this co-incidence; I just had to buy it and post the book to my son.

Since Scott was so interested in old cooking recipes, I looked through one of my old cookbooks from the early 1960's, one which I often turned to in order to produce some of our family favourite culinary delights.

I then trawled the internet for a similar copy to forward to my son in Australia, as a surprise. The only book available just happened to be in the next village where my son lives, in the Australian outback. I am always taken aback at such synchronistic happenings.

Last summer, Mike and I decided to de-clutter our loft, when inside one of the boxes I found a collection of old letters I had received from my Italian pen-friend during the 1960's. We had corresponded for fourteen years, throughout school, when Francesco went into the army, then he met and married Sofia and had baby Matteo. By this time, I too was married with two young sons.

After Mike and I had spent a pleasurable hour reading through those letters, renewing our memories, I kept a few photos, a hand painted Christmas card made by Sofia and their marriage announcement. On impulse, I wrote a letter and sent two copies, one to Francesco's last known address and the other to Francesco's family home, in the hope one of the messages would arrive safely after a lapse of forty-six years.

The following week, our daughter came to visit us and she was fascinated to hear about my pen-friend, with whom I had been communicating with, long before she was born and so she directly began researching for information on the internet. She found out that Sofia had qualified as an Art-Teacher, (like myself) and at sixty-three years old, had sadly passed away, just three weeks earlier.

I was shocked about this news because I had posted my two letters just one week earlier, not being aware of this situation. My daughter suggested I send my condolences to Francesco, via the Head Teacher of Sofia's school. However, it appears she now had a different family name, so may have divorced Francesco and re-married Gino, but the correspondence was re-directed to their son Matteo.

During September, I received a letter from Francesco, replying to my original letter, with no mention of the tragic news of his ex-wife but mentioning he divorced in the 1980's and that he too had re-married a lovely lady called Martina. My friend had a quadruple heart by-pass in the previous July, this was at the same time of Sofia's passing. I then presumed he may not have known about what had happened because he was seriously ill in hospital at the same time. It was only then I realised the family must have protected Francesco from the sad news, and yet I had sent my condolences in a following letter.

Only later have I been told that Martina had with-held my correspondence until Francesco was well enough to hear such sad news because he was asking questions about my family which I had sent in earlier letters. He wrote to tell me it was my letter which gave him the sad news about Sofia and he was very interested to know how I knew, before he did.

How extraordinary that I, someone from the distance past, should be the bearer of such news, when the family were hiding the truth. Were the 'other side' wanting me to tell my friend, or maybe it was Sofia wanting me to intervene? Is this synchronicity playing such a part?

Throughout my life there have been many synchronistic events, when I have not always understood their meaning, but it all made sense sometime later. Only last week, I had made arrangements to meet up with two friends, (on two consecutive days) from my past, one from my school days and the other from my first place of work. I had not seen those friends for between fifty-five and sixty years so I was uncertain whether we would recognise each other but I was full of excitement and anticipation on spending time catching up on our lives.

Within five minutes of my first arranged date, I was very surprised to be stopped by another friend from the 1960's. As we quickly tried to catch-up on our family news, I was tugged on my arm by yet another school friend from the 1950's. We quickly exchanged contact details because I was aware of my original appointment, my friend waiting in a nearby cafe.

I was still reeling from those synchronistic meetings when, the next day, I arrived to see my school pal when another of our classmates was standing close by. We instantly recognised each other, even though it had been fifty-eight years since we last met. Needless to say, many hours passed as we caught up with our life's journeys. I thought this was an end to the coincidences but no, the very next day, I then received a surprise invitation, to attend an art workshop, with the theme of nature and science, (my personal art topic), being run by a retired teacher, now a practising artist. This person turned out to be my friend from thirty years ago, when we were at Teacher Training College together. Yet another coincidence? I still wonder why my friends had all congregated for us to meet up, all in the same week, even why my Italian pen-friend has rekindled our friendship, quite by accident, after fifty-five-year lapse too. Only time will tell the meaning of those synchronistic events.

Last year, while on holiday in Devon, I visited a beautiful Art Deco House. When inside one of the bedrooms, I was looking at some old tins and jars of 'Brylcream', (a favourite hair product used by gentleman to obtain glossy hair), soaps and a selection of cosmetics used in the 1920-30's, when a lady nearby commented how it reminded her of times past. We chatted about the popular perfume, 'Evening in Paris', (very difficult to obtain around the war years), and 'Californian Poppy' too, then we both said simultaneously, "June". We were both taken aback at mentioning this rare fragrance, since we had mentioned it at exactly the same time and this happened to be my Mum's very favourite perfume. What synchronicity for Judy, (the name of the lady I had just met), to mention the fragrance at exactly the same time?

As we reminisced about our childhood, Judy then confided in me saying she keeps seeing feathers and yet she feels she cannot talk to anyone because they may not understand about her observations. I then told her I also see feathers and butterflies too. As we continued to chat with ease, as we had so much in common, both being very emotionally close to our Mums', both Mum's had died before we had our daughters, Judy was living two hundred miles away from Devon, the place where we were chatting, now living in the same town where I attended school. Although this lady was a complete stranger, we hugged warmly before parting when I reminded her to keep positive thoughts in order to maintain high vibrations. What a special synchronistic meeting.

Other examples of synchronicity are as follows:

- When I have phoned a friend to enquire about her health, since she has terminal cancer, only to find she had just that minute mentioned my name.
- Sometimes, I am aware of friends checking their mail, waiting for me to write, but I maybe busy at the time, but I will make a mental note to get in touch as soon as possible.
- I have posted an e-card and instantly received an incoming mail from the same person, someone who rarely sends communications.
- One evening, I was chatting on the phone to my daughter, when I mentioned I had not heard from a certain friend for a long time, then, their mail pinged instantly into my inbox. My daughter and I giggled at the synchronicity.
- I have actually picked up our phone to call a tradesperson, when the very same fellow was already tapping out our phone number, just as the phone rang. This caught us both by surprise, followed by much laughter at such synchronicity.
- I was out shopping, deep in thought, thinking about the pending Textiles exam and how fresh Irises would be a good subject for the observational drawing section. I then walked past two more shops and there, in the centre of the shop window were two vases of Irises.
- Later, as I arrived home, I noticed our drive looked untidy and so I made a mental note to ask Mike to weed and jet wash our drive. Once inside the house,

I sat down with a drink to make a 'job-list' just as I heard a soft knock at the door. It **was a fellow asking** if I would like my drive jet-washed.

- Following my Master's Degree, I was invited to exhibit in the National Gallery in Beijing, China. It was then necessary for me to communicate to the Director of the Museum in preparation for the forthcoming event. In the meantime, my Chinese friend Yan, had returned to Beijing and was working for a publishing company. Following yet another job move, she then secured a position at the National Gallery and one of her first tasks was to translate **my** letter.

- One time, I was writing to my cousin when, I do not know why but 'out of the blue', I mentioned our Grandma's date of death. I knew it was March 1937 but not the actual day. Unbeknown to me, my husband was down stairs, in our dining room, where he had picked up my Grandma's Family Bible, quite unawares of to whom I was writing or about the topic of my mail. Mike entered the room where I was writing and said, "Your Grandma died on the 15th March 1937". I did not know he had been reading Grandma's Bible, looking at the family birth and death section, just at the same time I was writing to my cousin. I was now able to forward the correct full date of death of our Grandma to my cousin.

- Mike and I decided to have some time-out together so we visited a nearby market town to saunter around the shops. Within about twenty minutes of arriving at the market, I said we needed to get in touch with his cousin because it had been almost a year since we last met, but maybe leave it until her daughter has returned to university. The next shop we entered, there was Mike's cousin and her daughter, just like magic, since we had not spoken on the phone for such a long time and certainly had not made any pre-arranged time to meet up. In fact, after several drinks, followed by a meal and a marathon six hour catch-up, this surely was synchronicity at its best.

- One Monday morning I received two text messages at 10.20am, one from each of my sons, who happen to live 12,000 miles apart. This is not the first time the three of us have linked up simultaneously.

- During breakfast, I mentioned to Mike that I had not heard from our German friend, Hans, playing in a Jazz band for more than forty-five years with my brother, who has since passed away. I had a feeling that Hans was missing the three longstanding band members, who had also passed.

  Our post then arrived, with a letter from Hans, explaining his recent hospital stay due to a serious heart operation. I just knew he had been contemplating on his own mortality and that of his close friends.

- On learning of my son in Australia had just become 'grain-free' and of his plans for a weekend away, I sent a text message for him not to drink beer but cider and wine instead.

  He immediately texted to say he had just at that moment bought cider and wine.

It is wonderful to have constant reassurance that we are connected to each other, no matter the distance.

- I needed to send a mail to my friend, Yvonne, but I did not have her e-mail address, only her phone number. As I was about to dial her number, my phone rang. It was my friend's husband. Yvonne wanted my e-mail address. There was much laughter at the synchronicity but if I had just phoned a second earlier, then our phones would have been engaged, as we were ringing each other for exactly the same information.

- Early last year, Mike and I went for a walk to Attingham Park, Shrewsbury, to see the winter snowdrops. (This is an hours drive from our home).
  Due to the cold weather, we scurried to the café for a hot drink but other walkers also had the same idea. The café was full and I had difficulty finding a seat but after several circuits of the large room, I was drawn to grey haired lady and asked if she minded us joining her table.
  As we sat with this couple, the conversation flowed, with lots of laughter for more than an hour. It was only as we parted that Margaret, mentioned she used to work for the Fire Service, sending out the engines. I then said Mike used to be a Fireman at our local town called Bloxwich, when Ben said he too had been in the Fire Service at Bloxwich, on the very same Red Watch. After further enquiries, it transpired that Mike and Ben were working in the same team although there were ten-year age difference and it had been forty-seven years since they had last seen

each other. Identification was made more difficult due to the thick scarf wrapped around Ben's chin and a woolly hat pulled down over his face.

After much hilarity and further reminiscing about past times, we have now exchanged contact details.

It never ceases to amaze me how this unseen connection happens and how I was drawn toward Margaret within a room full of strangers.

- During one of the times our son was visiting us, I asked him to please go into our loft and bring down a box full of my deceased brothers paperwork. I wished to start to declutter, but while sorting through the documents, I came across the 'Bill of Sale' of my brother's Lotus, car, which was garaged in Germany, some six years earlier, at the time of my brother's death.

  Our son looked on the internet to find out what happened to his Uncle's car, only to find it had only just been sold and it had now been brought back to the UK.

  It had been six years since we had looked at those documents and so it was yet another wonderful example of synchronicity. I have wondered whether my brother had given me a 'prompt' from over the other side about his beloved car.

  This is yet another occasion when I have a received a 'prompt' from the other side, so it appears this contact and communications continues wherever we are.

- Years ago, I often used to take an apple pie to my dear friend.

Last week, I was out shopping, when on impulse, I bought an apple pie and delivered it to my aged friend. She was shocked to see the contents of my bag because she had recently been reminiscing about those delicious pies. I guess I must have picked up her 'request', yet again. My daughter often uses this method if she needs something. She says it's fun to place an order.

- I was writing on this book about synchronicity and how we are all connected when I thought about my friend Mia. This is someone I used to work with in the early sixties, becoming firm friends, attending each other's wedding, meeting up when we had our children, but then lost touch when Mia moved house and area.
It had been forty years lapse since we last chatted and so on impulse, I phoned my friend. When she picked up the phone, Mia was in shock to hear my voice. Not due to the time span but because at that very moment, she was looking at a photo of us together, taken at her wedding in 1968. Mia had decided to send the photo, as a surprise, together with a letter, following a spate of decluttering, due to an imminent house move. How lovely to have constant examples of how we are all connected in this universal intelligence and just as I was writing about synchronicity too.

Chapter 6

Premonitions

Not only are we able to recall memories of past times, or even many early memories of our present life, but I have, on a few occasions, had a fleeting premonition about simple things, like telling my husband to be aware of incidents or traffic lights which are out of view at the time. Needless to say, this has proved very useful advice at the time.

One time, in the 1920's, when my Mum was a young woman living at home, she recalled a dream she had had that previous night to the family, as they sat around the Sunday breakfast table. The dream was about her travelling down a country lane, turning a corner then coming across some high metal gates. Behind the gates was a majestic old great stone building, a Convent.

After breakfast, as was customary on a Sunday, my Uncle used to drive my Grandparents, Aunts and Mum, together with the family dog, on various outings into the countryside for a picnic. Before setting off, my Uncle studied the maps and decided to travel in a part of the countryside where they had not previously ventured.

My Mum said everyone was chatting away in the car, when suddenly the surroundings became very familiar to her. She started to give directions to her brother to continue down the lane, around the corner and there stood the large ornate metal gates, standing in front of the Convent, just as my Mum had described her dream, earlier that morning, over breakfast. Everyone sat in silence for a long time as my Uncle confirmed he had never before driven the family in that part of the country. It was a new venture for all of them, since it was highly unlikely in the 1920's to have travelled far from their home town, other than by train. Not many people even owned a car during those times. In fact, my Dad was eighteen years old when he first saw the sea, thinking it was like a vast lake. This experience was on another occasion, when he was invited to take a trip with my Mum's family, in the car to the seaside.

Even when dreaming, there may-be some connection with a future event too. For example, I was on holiday in Germany, when I dreamt, I was in a clinic, having an injection. A few hours after my dream, I was having breakfast when the whole crown of my tooth fell out. Within an hour, I was in a clinic, having an injection in preparation for a temporary fix for my tooth. I had almost pre-empted this happening in my dream.

Recently, Mike and I visited one of our favourite cafes for a quiet cup of coffee. The din inside was unusually noisy, so much so, I put my fingers in my ears to deaden the sound since I have acute hearing. Mike, who has limited hearing, also found it too noisy for him.

On our way home, he bought a newspaper and as I opened the pages, there, inside was a double page spread about the noise in restaurants, while accompanying the script, was a photo of a lady with her fingers in her ears, just as I had done, earlier that morning. Yet another premonition.

A few years ago, I made our usual visit to a local farm, to collect our weekly vegetables, when I suggested to Mike for us to pop into the farm's coffee shop. I then commented the assistant was rather slow and not as efficient as the one who used to work there three years earlier.

On our way out of the cafe, there stood the fair-haired lady I had been talking about, the efficient one. On impulse, she had made an unexpected visit to the farm, in order to surprise the staff. These sorts of premonitions are beginning to happen with more regularity in my life.

Following my retirement from teaching six years earlier, I was discussing the talents of one of my gifted students with a few neighbours, when I actually found out old photographs of this girls stunning work. I had not thought about or mentioned this pupil during those past six years, when I received a message from my old school, that very same day, explaining that my ex-pupil, (the one whose work I had been looking at), had now been nominated for the Best Actress Award at the Globe Theatre in London. I was so proud of her achievement and also acknowledged the synchronicity of looking at the student's past work, after all those years, just as she was being considered for such a prestigious award.

I know I have had problems to solve within my artwork, when during the night, the answers are easily facilitated. It is as if our intuition works so much better when we are quieter and not distracted by every day interruptions.

The above accounts are just a few examples of precognition in operation and it never ceases to amaze me just how closely linked our energies are with each other and our surroundings. It is as if this built-in system is never turned off, because it acts as a constant support system for us.

Throughout this book, I have tried to give just a few examples to show just how we are all linked together, no matter how far away, the connection is never broken. This is why it is so important to love and ton be kind to each other because we are just a sum of the total whole. We are just a grain of sand on the beach and yet no matter how large or small, we are all part of this beautiful complex universe, constantly swirling in a state of flux.